Casting Your Troubles Into the Grand Canyon

By Matt Landry

Other titles from Matt Landry:

Learning to Be Human Again

Forward, Upward, Onward

Simply Happy

Introduction

"Let's get one thing straight," she said. "The Grand Canyon doesn't care how important, rich, poor, or beautiful you are. We're all the same in the Canyon's eyes."

She was answering a question I had asked about the kind of employees who worked in the Grand Canyon National Park's food concessions and gift shops. She sounded both annoyed and rushed.

It was nearly twenty years ago, and I recall the job interview had gone well. But I thought it unusual that someone would consider hiring an employee located almost 2,000 miles away, solely based upon a single, quick phone conversation. I was in Massachusetts, looking for a job in Arizona.

At the end of the phone call she abruptly announced, "I'd like to offer you a position. I'll get the paperwork ready and mail it out to you this afternoon. We can take it from there."

"Wait!" I blurted out before she could hang up. "I'd like a day or two to think about it. I mean, it's a big decision. A pretty big move, you know."

There was an uncomfortable pause. "Okay," she finally said. "Most either want to work here or they don't. They know that even before the interview. That's why they applied." There was a brief, awkward pause before she continued. "Get back to me in a day or two. I like you, I think you'd do okay here."

I hung up the phone and sighed. I had just been offered a job to work and live at the Grand Canyon for a season or two. My idea of a dream career wasn't selling cheap key rings and t-shirts at a gift shop for minimum wage, but I mean, it was the Grand Canyon. As any good realtor would exclaim, "It's all about location, location, location."

I phoned a friend, Brian, who knew someone who had worked at the Grand Canyon a few years before, doing similar work. I called him that afternoon, right after the interview to see if I could pick his brain.

Brian knew exactly who I was talking about. "You mean Carl? He worked there a few years ago. Yeah, I'd be happy to ask him. I know the job isn't what you think it is, though. I mean, like any job, it had its ups and downs from what I remember him saying."

"I understand, Brian. But I'd really like to get the inside scoop on what it's like to work there. My brain is telling me that it's an obvious opportunity right now, but my gut is telling me otherwise."

Brian called back the next day with the full report from the former Canyon employee, Carl.

"So, what's the story?" I asked. "Give it to me straight."

"Well," Brian said, "here's what I found out. Carl said most of it was pretty routine, but the turnover rate was pretty high. A lot of the employees came from all walks of life. Many were retired. Some were foreign workers who wanted to experience what they thought the United States was like. A few college kids worked there during their summer break. Everyone lives in a dormitory setting. They share rooms, usually in pairs, so pray you get a good roommate. Not as many outdoorsy types as you'd think work there. He said there was a recurring theme with many of the people there though. Not just employees either. A lot of the visitors, too."

"And what's that?" I asked.

Brian took a moment, obviously trying to figure out

how to explain what Carl had told him. "He said, and I'm still trying to wrap my head around this because it doesn't make sense to me, that there were a lot of folks there that went way beyond just having an adventurous or cool job. They just wanted to end their suffering and confusion by somehow casting their troubles into the Grand Canyon, hoping that it would accept them and, in turn, heal their pain."

Brian seemed perplexed by that statement. Baffled by the whole concept.

I, on the other hand, knew exactly what it meant.

I declined the job.

CHAPTER ONE

Casting Your Troubles into the Grand Canyon

"I can still remember my first experience of standing at the edge of the Grand Canyon and looking into it. It was so awesome, it took a fair amount of restraint to prevent me from jumping into it, because I was certain I could fly."

–Mark Goulston

The Grand Canyon is vast, to say the least. When we refer to enormity, the Canyon is often used to describe something unusually large, as if nothing gets any bigger than the Grand Canyon.

"It was almost as big as the Grand Canyon ..."

"Wow. That big? That's big!"

The Grand Canyon is a place of both awe and mystery. It has been to me, anyway.

My first visit to what many may call the ultimate Mecca of vacation destinations was in the early 1990s. I was doing an exciting trip across the United States with a friend. We were in our early 20s and hadn't been many places outside New England. In many ways this was our first real taste of true freedom as young adults. The timing just happened to take us there on the Fourth of July, and on a weekend. To say it was busy is an understatement.

I can remember my first sighting of the enormous gap in the Earth from what I think was Mather Point—an extremely popular, accessible location to see that expansive Canyon in all its glory. Regardless of the exact location, it took my breath away. I mean, absolutely took it away. I didn't realize something like that existed.

Well, I mean I did, but to see it up close and in person is hard to describe. Impossible, really.

That first road trip across the States was

memorable for so many reasons. One of them was the preparation. Since it was before the days of the internet and cell phones, I had mailed postcards to the tourist departments of all the states we intended to travel through. One by one their responses arrived and, like a little kid, I excitedly looked forward to whichever one would arrive in the mailbox each day.

By the time I had finished with it, Arizona's travel brochure was well worn and dog-eared.

The Grand Canyon was high on the list of must-sees. Without much knowledge of what was out there, my only frame of reference included things like the Brady Bunch's road trip in their big station wagon, and Bugs Bunny and his suitcase full of stickers of the places he had been: Mt. Rushmore, the Hoover Dam, Niagara Falls, and the Grand Canyon. Those were the places I was familiar with. In many ways, that was America to me. Route 66, left turns at Albuquerque, and for some reason, Graceland. I needed to see Graceland. (And we did, thank you, thank you very much.)

We didn't stay long at the canyon lookout. We had a deadline to make it to Las Vegas by nightfall. As a matter of fact, now that I think of it, many of my photos of the Grand Canyon on that trip were taken from the car window. It was so busy that there was no parking anywhere. This was before the new visitor's center was constructed and the shuttle buses arrived to easily transport tourists about. It was all either by car, if you could park, or foot. Nothing else.

Even with all the rushed commotion, the Canyon hooked me. Actually, it was my first trip through the desert that had hooked me. The Grand Canyon reeled me in without a fight of any kind after that. There was an energy there that went beyond the landscape. For some it's the ocean or a lake, for others it's the mountains. I love both, but for me it was the Southwest desert and specifically, the Grand Canyon. It was home to me. There is an indescribable solace and peace to be found there.

You either get the desert, or you don't. Many would view the lack of color and trees as barren. I see life there, everywhere. I see the history of a Native American nation before the European settlers arrived. I see the promise of a new country in the brave pioneers who risked their lives for a better life. I see a bigger sense of freedom, both physically and mentally, than you find in places like the Northeast United States.

I was unaware that you could go to the bottom of the Canyon. It just seemed so impossible. I assumed its walls were unassailable and went straight down to the bottom, like, well, a giant canyon. As time passed, I would hear stories of people taking mules to the bottom. I assumed the trip took months, sort of like a Lewis and Clark thing with salted fish and a fifty-pound sack of flour for supplies. Little did I know that there was an air-conditioned store that served cold beer down there. There were even heated cabins for guests.

I would visit the Grand Canyon and the desert many, many more times. The lure was strong, and I wasn't sure why. It was more than just the tourist attraction we've all come to know. As I noted, it had become a place of refuge and solace for me.

On another memorable visit, I witnessed something I'll never forget. Standing on Mather Point and leaning against the railing were a dozen or so folks with paper bags over their heads. They had been led to the Canyon's edge that way—their vision blocked by brown paper. After a countdown, the bags were removed, and each of those people saw the Grand Canyon for the first time in a dramatic unveiling. Everyone at the point felt the collective sense of awe. Can you imagine seeing the Canyon for the first time that way?

The rim was a safe place to observe it all. With the warnings against hiking to the bottom, I assumed that going to the lowermost point, especially by foot, was impossible. Only experienced, adventurous, athletic types did that. I imagined those slippery walls along the way, with Sherpas and rope necessary to accomplish the feat.

CHAPTER TWO

Where Does Life Begin

and Where Does it End?

Where does life begin and where does it end?

I'm not necessarily referring to the actual years of breath we take or the moment of conception or birth. I'm talking about the life we live.

When people pass away and the gravestone is carved and erected, there's a name and a date. The numbers, the years etched on the granite, indicate the amount of time they spent on Earth. The most important and overlooked part of that date is the dash between them. What I want to know is, How good was your dash? How was it spent? How did you spend your time?

I want to know how meaningful *my* dash will be. What did I do? How did I act and react? How much time was wasted? How much did I love? Did I make the best of it?

"We live in a wonderful world that is full of beauty, charm and adventure. There is no end to the adventures that we can have if only we seek them with our eyes open."

–Jawaharlal Nehru

After muddling through a major depression as I approached turning forty, that dash became even more important.

For many, depression is a lot of things. Less lust for life would be a great overall description. Food doesn't taste as good, events and people that once produced peace or joy no longer do. Depression is exactly how it sounds: Things are almost pushed in or pushed down. Many parts of life are less likely to hold importance. Showering, eating, and for some, living.

Another major factor behind a depression is regret. What a useless emotion regret is: looking to the past and wallowing in your misery based upon what you did and the things you wish you had done. Much of it is based upon accomplishment. Most of it is just useless wallowing in the past and feeling sorry over making often-necessary mistakes.

"I wish I had saved more money, asked her (or him) out on a date, bought the house, took the trip, or become more successful. If only I had ... I really should have ..."

When I went through that depression, the nights were unbearable. Long, sleepless, and filled with anxiety. I didn't know where I was going, and I was ashamed of where I had been. Regret has a way of dragging you into a pit that's sometimes tough to climb out of. It seems silly now, looking back on it. Putting so much value on the things in the past that had already happened and I had no control over.

But, there was light in the midst of all of it. Life had tapped me on the shoulder and said, "You know those things you've avoided? The things that you should have taken care of a long time ago? The growing up you needed to do but didn't want to? Yeah, we're here for a visit now. All at once. We need to talk."

Apparently, denying a problem or stuffing away emotions and trauma doesn't make them disappear.

It hit me like a freight train with all the trappings of what a proper depression brings: self-loathing, hopelessness, worthlessness, jealousy, loneliness, sadness, and anger. I had been a victim of my own doing. I wanted an easy life, but in striving for one, I had created my own monster that needed to be addressed.

And so I did what I should have done a long time before. I addressed it. I pulled up those truths I had ignored and laid them on the table. I went through them one at a time and gave them the proper attention they deserved. I loved them and thanked them for their hard-earned lessons.

Then I moved on.

I found that I had control of the future I wished for. I just had to start creating it. I needed to do some difficult work. I needed to stop looking back and begin to move forward. The only permission I gave myself for looking back was to see how far I had come.

So, back to the original question. Where does your

life begin and where does it end?

To try and answer that, I can say from personal experience that you really begin to *truly* live when you can look fear in the eye and brush it aside. This fear can be a host of things. It's not all the same for everyone. For some it's heights, snakes, hurricanes, or public speaking. Others are plagued by some deeper and longer-lasting fears. Financial security, health, success, living up to a parent's standards. Death of a loved one. Their own mortality.

I didn't know what I was scared of. I suspect it was success. I always played the role of the humble man, but that was just a cover for not accomplishing much. I rolled my eyes at people who drove BMWs and made good money or accomplished great things to cover up my own inadequacies.

The biggest lesson I learned through the maturing process during my depression was in fact that I created my own life. I was in charge. Where I was or what I had become in life was nobody else's responsibility or fault. I was self-centered, immature, and impatient. I lacked discipline and grit, and I was hypersensitive.

I no longer regret any of these character traits.

They led me to who I am today. This wasn't anyone's responsibility but mine. It wasn't my parents' fault, or the government's, or my teachers', bosses', or friends'. It was all me.

As part of the healing process, I needed to not just discover who I really was. I had to re-create myself. I had to take the old me apart and put him back together again piece by piece. Attitude, morals, kindness, success, goals, hopes, dreams. One by one I dug in the dirt and planted new character traits and mental fortitude. Then I watered and fed those good parts and weeded out the bad.

"The challenge of life, I have found, is to build a résumé that doesn't simply tell a story about what you want to be, but it's a story about who you want to be."

–Oprah Winfrey

There's something about the decade markers of our lives—turning thirty, forty, fifty—that seems to throw everyone for a contemplative loop. After beginning to re-create myself after depression, I accomplished a lot as a person in the decade from age forty onward. I created a more optimistic mindset and an improved attitude. I had better tools and experience to help my mental health along.

As I approached my fiftieth birthday, I knew that I didn't want to go through another depressive state. So I decided that I was going to climb the forty-eight 4,000-foot peaks of New Hampshire by the time I turned fifty.

This was not an exclusive goal or adventure by any means. Lots of people have done it. But to me, it was like hiking Everest. I was a pretty avid hiker who had done many of the peaks previously, but I had never kept track of what I had climbed and when. So I took on this goal as if I had never climbed any of them at all.

I was about forty-seven when I started.

I'll cut to the chase. I finished them with time to spare and wept like a child the day after the last one. If you'd like to read about that adventure, I wrote a book about it called *Forward, Upward, Onward*. As a personal celebration of the event, I released the book on my fiftieth birthday.

I'm not belittling the achievement by any means. It

was hundreds of miles and thousands and thousands of feet of elevation gain. It's hard work, time-consuming, and not all fun and games.

"One who gains strength by overcoming obstacles possesses the only strength which can overcome adversity."

–Albert Schweitzer

When you finish the forty-eight peaks, there's an application you can fill out to receive a patch and scroll from the Appalachian Mountain Club indicating that you climbed all the summits. They also hold a pizza banquet in a big high school auditorium to honor those who finished the goal and present that fancy scroll .

The event was a last-minute attendance for me. I didn't need the scroll, personally. I finished the goal for other reasons. But I'm glad I went.

Just before the scrolls were handed out, they ran a slideshow showcasing photos submitted by folks who had finished their peaks the previous year. The slides rolled and music played behind them.

The show evolved to a part that displayed reasons why so many had done the forty-eight 4,000-footers goal over time and finally accomplished them.

I had cancer. I didn't know if I was going to live. The mountains reminded me about what it was like to really live.

My wife left me. It was the most traumatic time of my life. The mountains healed me.

I lost my job. I didn't have anywhere else to turn. The mountains took me in.

My father never completed them and regretted it. He has since passed away. I finished them for him.

That part shook me to my core, because I had also had a much bigger why behind the reasons for doing it. The goal was hard, and it needed to be hard for it to change me. Something usually needs to be hard to change you. Many would say that's what hiking does. It heals and changes you through the challenge it offers, both physically and mentally.

Much of the enjoyment of completing a hard task or goal is the process, although it often doesn't feel like it at the time. It's finding out what you're made of. It's grit, determination, and stamina. Much like those old travel brochures I had mailed away for all those years ago, the fun was in the planning and mental adventure.

The trip was fun. But the planning, flipping through the pages of endless possibilities, may have been even more fulfilling than the trip itself.

Doing things that are hard or, in some cases, seem impossible is a great way to confront your fears or the limitations you put on yourself. It's coming out of your shell to test the limits of your capabilities. It's thinking you can't, then realizing that your head and thoughts often lie to you.

I think that's why hiking is such a good tool against mental illnesses like depression. We have a sort of script in our heads that runs all day long, almost on automatic. It often repeats, *I'm not good enough, smart enough, or beautiful enough. I suck. That's impossible. I could never do or accomplish that.*

The script reminds us of our lacks and limitations over and over again. But do you know what I learned? The script is bullshit. It's lying to us on a regular basis. That's why it's important to do things that we don't think we can accomplish. To set lofty goals and keep aiming for the stars.

That's why hiking is an important ally in my fight to remain optimistic. It's taught me that I'm capable of doing things I never thought I could do.

"While on top of Everest, I looked across the valley towards the great peak Makalu and mentally worked out a route about how it could be climbed. It showed me that even though I was standing on top of the world, it wasn't the end of everything. I was still looking beyond to other interesting challenges."

–Sir Edmund Hillary

People who achieve a hard goal often say the same thing: It's pure bliss upon completing it. But then comes the crash. You think to yourself, *Now what*? There's an uncomfortable pause brought about by not having something to aspire to anymore. The goal was hard, it was achieved. Now what's next?

That thought stuck with me a few months after the glow of hiking the forty-eight summits wore off. There are other hiking lists and goals to accomplish in the Northeast. The hundred highest, the sixty-seven 4,000-foot peaks, the fifty-two with a view. Some do the forty-eight all over again in a certain season (winter is the hardest). Some even go after something called The Grid. That's hiking all forty-eight peaks in every month of the year. (That's 576 peaks total, in case you needed the math.)

None of those appealed to me. The mountains of New Hampshire burned me out. It was like a loving mother asking her son to leave home. To go out and explore new territory and adventures. To leave the nest, so to speak.

When I was a young boy, we used to frequent the White Mountain region in New Hampshire. It was a cheap, accessible vacation destination for us. We would often walk a long-abandoned train trestle that could almost be called the rail trail of its day. At the end of the three-mile walk, we took a left up a short trail to Franconia Falls. It's a great, natural water slide that provided us with large, flat rocks to lie upon, or the running stream in front to swim in. As I grew older and got my driver's license, some of the first trips I took were back to that region and invariably back to the three-mile walk up the flat path, then the left one back to Franconia Falls.

At the end of the Trestle Trail, instead of taking the left, you could follow the trail over a bridge and continue. At the time, this was called the Wilderness Trail. In all the times I ever visited there, I never crossed that bridge. Not once. That bridge, whether I knew it or not, was like a symbol for the unknown. It represented places I was not supposed to go to and things I wasn't supposed to see. It was where true, experienced explorers dared to go.

When I completed the last peak of the 4,000-footers goal, the final one, I finally crossed over that symbolic bridge, both going over it and returning, having seen all that could be seen from the other side. Some of the most incredible views and experiences in all of those mountains lay just beyond that bridge. I saw it. Finally. At age forty-nine I had become that fearless explorer who, in my younger eyes, could dare to visit such difficult and dangerous lands.

Originally, in my mind people who ventured out there never came back. I wasn't totally wrong. The person who ventures to places like that fades away, and a much different person often comes back.

CHAPTER THREE

By the Way, You're Hiking to the Bottom of the Grand Canyon ...

One day, as if the Universe was listening, it tapped me on the shoulder. The answer to what my next task or lesson or challenge or whatever it was I needed should be simply presented itself.

"You have to hike to the bottom of the Grand Canyon," it said.

It wasn't like the clouds parted, or bushes burned, or anything like that. It was more of an obvious feeling. I just knew it was the next right thing to do. Just like the 4,000-footers, it just felt right.

You need to see what's at the bottom. Just like the bridge you needed to cross in the White Mountains to help complete yourself, you need to wander down and see what's there.

The feeling also implied that instead of casting my troubles into the Grand Canyon, I needed to personally take them down to the bottom myself. They needed to be hand-delivered and caringly placed at the Colorado River to be floated away, or whatever happened to them when they reached the bottom.

It's almost like I thought that casting my troubles from the canyon rim could pose some issues. They could blow away or end up on a trail somewhere, or worse, hit someone in the face on the way down. Maybe they were like a flu that would pass in front of someone who would inherit or catch those problems.

No, I thought, *I'd better deliver them myself to make sure they arrive safely.*

"I believe in evolution. But I also believe, when I hike the Grand Canyon and see it at sunset, that the hand of God is there also."

–John McCain

In order to hike to the bottom of the Grand Canyon and stay overnight, reservations are required. These permits are difficult to get, but for some reason, I knew I would be granted one.

I was right. Just like an expected gift at Christmas, the email arrived to say: "Welcome. We've been waiting for you."

I felt I needed to stay overnight because it's about a sixteen-mile round-trip hike. I wasn't worried about going down. My concern was coming back up.

Unlike the New Hampshire mountains I was accustomed to, the terrain here was reversed. When you hike a mountain, the hard and slow part is generally on the way up. You're gaining elevation and walking uphill. Although the descent can be difficult, it's usually the quicker and easier of the two. Walking to the bottom of the Grand Canyon, on the other hand, posed the opposite scenario.

The easier walk down occurs first and the hard trek up comes after. Signs at most of the Grand Canyon trailheads state; "Hiking down is optional. Hiking up is mandatory." A warning for the multitudes of folks who start down for a day trip and think: *This isn't too bad. Maybe I'll go just a bit*

exhausted. This time, we decided to fly into Vegas and stay in Laughlin, Nevada. It's a sleepy but pleasant little gambling town situated on the Colorado River, about ninety minutes outside Las Vegas. The people are friendly, the rooms are cheap, and the beer is cold.

The next morning, we headed out early for the three-and-a-half-hour ride into the park. We were able to see the sun slowly rise on the horizon on the drive in. I love catching sunrises in the Southwest. We rarely get to see great ones in places like Massachusetts because trees and buildings block them. When you have open territory in front of you, like the desert affords, it makes them that much better.

We pulled into a small market just outside the park and re-stocked some supplies and food for the hike. We went simple. Peanut butter and bagels, a few candy bars, and lots of water.

We arrived at the park and prepared peanut butter-bagel sandwiches in the parking lot. We filled water bottles and re-fitted and re-adjusted our packs for the trip down.

In some ways I was nervous. I'm not sure why. I guess that I often don't think of myself as a hiker who has a lot of mileage and knowledge under his belt.

It reminds me of a story from the year before. A group of friends and I were planning a moderate hike in Maine. After looking at the details of the fairly average hike, I announced that it looked like it was for experienced hikers. Rolling his eyes, one friend calmly replied, "YOU are an experienced hiker, knucklehead." Apparently I keep forgetting about that part.

We chose to hike a loop to the canyon floor, then back up the next day. Down South Kaibab, up Bright Angel Trail. Both are well-traveled and well-worn paths.

The pathway that leads down on the South Kaibab trail is essentially a giant ramp. There were times I thought you could probably drive a car out there on some sections. It was certainly a big difference from the rocks and roots of New Hampshire.

I often find my hikes in the Northeast fulfilling, but most of them are spent looking down, concentrating on where my next step will be.

There's a different rhythm to a hike in New Hampshire or the Appalachian range in general.

You're choosing which rocks to step on, and where your foot placement should be in order to make it all work well. It's like a well-choreographed ballet with the strategy of a chess game. You start to think about the step after the next, with the current step having already been thought of.

In other words, because of the terrain, you need to think about not only where you're stepping, but the step placement after that. Rock hopping can be fun, but mentally challenging.

Your subconscious thoughts are a constant narration of, *If I step here with my left foot, my right can push up on that rock. Is that root slippery? It looks slippery. Wet rock there, step on the dry ...*

When I think of hiking, walking in the outdoors is obvious, but I directly equate it to those obstacles. Rocks, roots, rain, ice, boulders, slides, trees, you name it. It's both mental and physical.

The Canyon is much different. It affords something I don't normally get to do: methodically walk. In many ways, I could set my pace and walking in the Canyon to a metronome. Step ... step ... step ... I like this rhythm for a couple of different reasons. For one, I can stop thinking so much and just let my thoughts flow. Second, I can enjoy the scenery around me much more.

When you hike in the White Mountains, your gaze remains mostly down, looking for those roots and rocks. When you're walking without obstructions, like in the Grand Canyon, you can look up at the world around you. You can notice the changing environment and geology. You can really take in the overall scenery.

As we headed down on South Kaibab, the vast space around us was difficult to comprehend. The rim faded behind us as we continued downward. It was like floating in the middle of an ocean bursting with reds and browns. It made me feel the same way I feel staring at the stars on a moonless summer night, wondering where I come from and what the hell the meaning of all of this is. As I walked, I somehow knew that I was in the hands of something bigger and more powerful than me. The Canyon was taking me in lovingly.

Nature heals. Science is just catching up to the research behind it, but being outside in all of its splendor and beauty is good for us in both the body and the soul. We connect with things that aren't concrete and steel, sawed and painted wood, or plaster. The air is fresher and cleaner. The spirit connects to something we can't always explain.

In my eyes, the whole Canyon is one. A living and breathing entity in all its parts and pieces. Mesas, trails, gradient colors of rock and sand. These are no different from a stomach, liver, lungs, and heart in a living being. All parts make the whole thing work together. Spirit included.

The Canyon has a soul just like a mountain or waterfall does.

As we rambled down, we passed several mule trains heading up and down. Guests up on their rides smiled and cheerfully greeted us. The wranglers who led the pack, dressed in classic cowboy attire, often just pinched the front rim of their cowboy hats with a gentle nod as they approached. I fully expected them to quietly utter, "Howdy."

We weren't rewarded with that gesture, but I said it in my head. It seemed good enough.

My eyes were drawn to the landscape around me as we descended. It looked much different than I had expected. The pace also felt much unlike what I thought it would be. The giant, ramp-like trail made for good walking, but it called for different leg muscles than I had predicted. Strolling down sounds easy enough, but I was fighting gravity. Instead of propelling myself forward, I was holding back, much like applying the brakes in a car going downhill.

The grade was gentle, and the path wound around and farther away from the rim after every step. Unlike my first impressions years before of sheer cliffs that went straight down to the canyon below, the trail inched and eased its way carefully and methodically from the top all the way down. There were many moments when it was difficult to see what lay beyond or behind us. At one such moment, we rounded a corner, and there it was before us, just as plain and welcoming as I would have imagined.

The Colorado River.

The winding path we were on led to a suspension bridge. Built in the 1920s, it held the same charm, history, and workmanship of the lodges and other structures along the rim. It crossed the Colorado River then disappeared into a tunnel on the other side. The craftsmanship of the whole spectacle, in what seemed the middle of nowhere, was impressive.

We crossed the bridge above the swirling water below. I stopped momentarily to look at the river from about the center of the bridge. This, to me, is the true bottom of the Canyon. It doesn't get any lower geographically than the river that created this masterpiece. The force that carved stone over thousands and millions of years. That chipped away layer after layer of silt, sand, and rock.

This flowing river was where I was supposed to find all those troubles that others before me had surrendered to the Canyon, troubles that had floated down from the rim. I think it was where I was meant to toss mine. It didn't feel like it, though. I looked, but I didn't see anyone else's troubles hanging around. Maybe the river had taken them away. Maybe it took them to the next destination, or to Moab, Utah, where the river continues on. Maybe the problems and troubles were in the river itself.

But it didn't look like it. It still looked like a plain river to me. The water swirled and rushed, but I didn't get the feeling that it was full of problems. It almost seemed too busy to care, actually. Making canyons is hard work, and the river is still doing that work. It didn't look like it wanted to take on the responsibility of people's troubles. It almost felt like in *The Wizard of Oz* when the wizard was exposed for who he really was. There was this big expectation of an all-powerful wizard, and all along he was just a traveling carnival schmuck behind a curtain.

The river is no schmuck, though. Its persistence and determination are impressive, to say the least. I mean, let's face it: It created the Grand Canyon. That alone is pretty remarkable. After years of erosion one inch at a time, it wore away the rock in its path. Over and over and over again. It just kept moving on. Still productive and doing its part for what its true intended purpose is: making canyons. Not accepting troubles.

We pushed ahead past the bridge and through the tunnel, then took a few moments to rest along the river in a sandy, almost beach-like area. My legs and feet were killing me as I dipped them into the cold water. The day was surprisingly warm and I already was starting to have trepidations and worries about the trek up the next day. I'm prone to heat stroke very easily and I was concerned about the shape of my legs.

We set up camp mid-day and walked to Phantom Ranch. It's basically a canteen that also has a small store with minimal merchandise for guests who venture to the bottom. I filled out and mailed two postcards for my niece and nephew. The cards would have a custom "Bottom of the Grand Canyon" postmark and be carried up by mule the next day. I thought the campy gifts were perfect and wouldn't be lost in translation. There was life below the rim.

There was also cold beer. After having perhaps the most refreshing one of those in my life, we started the short walk back to our tents at Bright Angel Campsite. Along the way, we encountered an inconspicuous, friendly guy with a scrubby beard and a focus in his eye. He casually asked us if and where there were any water sources nearby. I told him that we had one right at our campsite. So we arrived at the site together and parked ourselves at a picnic table for a few minutes. I asked if he had brought one of the mules down. He told us that he was doing a rim-to-rim-to-rim that day.

Doing a rim-to-rim-to-rim means that he started at the South Rim, hiked down, then up to the North Rim on the other side. Then he hiked back down and would be continuing back up the South Rim again, where he had started.

"All in one day?" I asked it casually, but my brain was going bananas trying to wrap my head around a guy, sitting in front of me, tackling over 12,000 feet of elevation gain and almost thirty miles of hiking in a single day.

"I am," he calmly replied as he looked down and filled his water bottle. "I started about three o'clock this morning, and I'll finish back up the South Rim this evening, probably by headlamp."

I was impressed. Not so much about the sheer feat in front of him, but more about the why behind what he was doing. I didn't ask. Sometimes the why is simply to test your physical limits. Most times your why is personal. I used to ask some of the thru-hikers on their way to finishing the 2,200-mile Appalachian Trail that same question, and I got some pretty insightful answers. This didn't seem the appropriate time to ask that question, though. I don't think he knew the answer himself.

After the intrepid rim-to-rim-to-rim hiker headed off, my friend and I ate dinner then unwound at the campsite to watch the day fade into night.

Holy cathedrals are not just contained in buildings of wood, stone, and glass. The element of God or the Universe is everywhere in the natural.

A place like the Grand Canyon reminds you of that. With all that vastness, it has a way of making you feel small, in a good way. It reminds you that there are things bigger than you. It takes the focus off of you.

The Canyon shifts in the light. Shadows deepen and retreat. It almost feels as though it were two separate places. I often get this feeling doing a hike at night. In the light, a mountain takes one form, and during the night it takes another. I imagine a city can give the same impression. I know Vegas is two very different places day to night.

There's little light pollution in and around the park, so you can see stars you've never seen before. It's a treat to see the Milky Way if you've never witnessed it. It's both astounding and humbling.

Seeing the sky full of countless, speckled stars makes you realize that the vastness of the Canyon is nothing in comparison to the Universe. The Grand Canyon is huge. But the Universe? Forget about it. When we realize that those stars are billions of miles away, with countless other planets a hundred times the size of Earth floating around out there, it makes you put things into perspective.

The world is a big place, and the Universe is even

bigger. We fuss and worry about nothing in the grand scheme of it all. Traffic, board meetings, and deadlines go out the window when we sit and contemplate the clouds or the stars. The outside human-made world goes away when we immerse ourselves in things much *bigger* than ourselves.

One of the benefits of a regular hiking regimen isn't the speed or mileage you climb. In my opinion, it's how you feel the next morning. It's the ability to tackle another mountain the day after a big hike.

I was hoping the pain would subside from the climb down and that the climb out of the Canyon would go as smoothly as possible. When I awoke the next morning, my legs were still killing me. *Shit, I thought, this is going to be a long, long walk today.* The stinging sunburn from the previous day's intense sun also made me think, *I hope the heat doesn't rise too high for the trip back up.*

I had reserved breakfast for us at Phantom Ranch and practically had to take out a mortgage to pay for it. *That coffee had better be incredible,* I thought. Turned out, it was well worth the cost. It had given us the peace of mind that we could have a nice, hot bite in a warm cafeteria and didn't have to haul extra food down or up for the trip. As it was, stuffed with a sleeping bag, tent, extra water, and clothing, my pack felt like the equivalent of carrying a small piano on my back.

We decided to take Bright Angel Trail back to the rim. It's one of the oldest and most used trails. From the campground, the trail crosses, then runs parallel to, the Colorado River for a little over a mile.

We crossed another suspension bridge to the other side of the river. Much like the bridge I had crossed a few years earlier in the White Mountains, this one held a similar charm. I now was the daring and fearless explorer who discovered that the trip wasn't nearly as frightening or intimidating as I had thought. Difficult, but far from impossible. We still had the hardest part to tackle, but we were ready.

The sight of the brown, swirling water was refreshing and calming. We hiked alone, with the trail to ourselves. You could hear the rush of the water against the riverbanks and rocks. I suddenly thought about how beautiful solitude can be, but in contrast, how it relates to the wonderful people I have come to know. *Just like a river makes little sound without the benefit of stones, we make little noise in the world without the benefit of other people,* I thought.

The walk up and back was refreshingly cool, bordering on cold. The entire trail followed along the shade of the canyon. My legs ached but started to loosen up as we went along. I insisted on a slow and steady pace, my preferred way to hike. Besides, we were in the Grand Canyon. Why would we ever want to rush this?

We slowly began to encounter more mules headed down and hikers coming up. Most passed us with wide grins and quicker paces. There were several rest stops and areas with more signs of life than a simple trail offers. One of them was the campground, Indian Garden. It's located about halfway up (or down) Bright Angel Trail, and several other trails intersected there as well.

Indian Garden and the whole surrounding area leading up to it were surprisingly lush with vegetation. Ferns, reeds, and trees swayed in the breeze as we walked through them. A creek runs through the location, supplying ample moisture for deep, leafy green plants along the trail. I almost felt at home, like I was hiking in the Northeast.

As we approached a trail intersection near the

campground, a man came walking towards us taking long, awkward strides. He looked lost. With blazing red hair, ill-fitting boots, and an oversized, gas station cowboy hat, he seemed about as out of place as a fart in church. "Is this the way to Colorado River?" he asked in a thick, what sounded like Scandinavian accent.

"It is," we replied. "Straight down that way, then left." We pointed him toward the trail we had just brought up.

"Thanks," he said, and off he awkwardly went.

People from all over the world are enamored with the United States, particularly the American West. For many reasons, it has the connotation of some of the last frontiers that were conquered in modern times. The spirit of the open spaces, snowcapped mountains, rugged and unforgiving landscape, and deep reds and browns of the sandstone and rock that encompass the area entice people from all over the world. I'd venture to guess that Coca-Cola, John Wayne, and Levi's jeans have a deeper connection with the Japanese now than with the people of the United States. I could be wrong, though.

It was obvious that we were getting closer to the

upper canyon. The surroundings were changing. The Canyon holds more treasures than its obvious outward majesty. It's also a time capsule of geology and the past. It's a simple map of floods, droughts, and civilizations come and gone. From the dinosaurs and the mammoths, to the Native Americans. I could see the various layers of stone indicating all of it in front of me. It was the history of millions of years.

We continued and held true to an earlier promise we had made between us that no matter what, we would be the beacon of encouragement and hope to anyone we met upon the trail. With broad, sometimes forced smiles, we kept at it one arduous step at a time. As we pressed on, the crowds on the trail started to become heavier. We were starting to reach the areas where day hikers venture down to say they had done part of the trail into the canyon. We were carrying full packs, sweat soaked shirts, and wore dirt-covered boots. Many of the folks we were encountering now were wearing fanny packs and flip-flops.

"You hiked to the bottom? That's crazy!" we heard a few say.

After several thousand feet of elevation gain and

well over six miles, the steps were getting harder and more painful. But I continued to hold true to a discovery I had made over thousands of miles of past hiking. It's a mantra that I repeated at the start of the hike that morning and also use often in life: *Each step may hurt, but each step is not impossible. Keep moving forward, one small step at a time, and you'll get to where you're going.*

We eventually made it to the rim and were promptly high-fived by our friend awaiting us. He had stayed in the park overnight, and seeing him at the finish was like coming home. Luckily the car was parked nearby. I simply wanted to put on a clean shirt and take the heavy pack off my back.

After a little cleaning up and a few laughs at the car, we gimped our way to Bright Angel Lounge to have a cold beer.

Strangely, after we had come up, we never looked behind us. Not once. The hike was done, but I guess the impact hadn't hit yet. Sitting at the bar, in the middle of a sip of beer, I turned to my friends and simply stated, "Dude. We just hiked the Grand Canyon."

"Strength doesn't come from what you can do. It comes from overcoming the things you once thought you couldn't."

–Rikki Rogers

Finally completing the Grand Canyon hike from rim to bottom and back again reminded me that we can all conquer whatever lies before us. It only takes one small step at a time. That's the way anything is tackled.

Once you start getting outside yourself and whatever your present life situation is, and face whatever lies before you, it becomes easier, as long as you do it moment to moment. No past, no future, just the present second you're in. You can't suffer the past or future because they don't exist. When you're suffering, most times it's nothing more than your memory and your imagination.

That's how hiking helped me. You'll eventually get to the summit or your destination if you just keep concentrating on the step you're taking, then the next, then the next. Stop thinking about the peak that lies before you and focus on the step in front of you instead. Most fears aren't lived in the moment; they're projected and magnified unrealistically. The same goes for a hundred other emotions.

With all of the emotions we have to deal with, how can we get them all straight? Jealousy, hate, anger, joy, happiness, sadness, anxiety, excitement. Who can keep track?

It's much easier than we think. There are only two categories that emotions fall into. Just two:

Love and fear. That's it.

When you come from a place of love, the world starts to come together. Not just the world collectively, but your own personal world starts to come together. Things make sense, the Universe starts to hand you things. It conspires to help you.

But when you come from a place of fear, then the mentality of lack rears its ugly head. "There's not enough." "I can't do it." "Why did I do it?" "This is impossible."

Facing fear eliminates fear. Facing it and even embracing it makes us realize that we can't outrun our problems or fears. They catch up to us. They hold us back, not only from success, but from being our best selves. People who love, give. It's just a natural byproduct of love and light, and they emit their light more.

"Work out your own salvation. Do not depend on others."

–Buddha

I had declined the job at the Grand Canyon years before because I knew damn well that I wouldn't be going there for the great outdoors. I was running away without facing my fears. I was hoping that, instead of doing the work, it could magically be done for me. I was trying to figure something out, but I wanted it to be figured out for me. I wanted to transfer the confusion and pain to another source.

Granted, there is often a time and a place for things that take us far away as a temporary form of escape. We use them all the time. Movies, food, drugs, social media, sex, smoking. These are all temporary moments when we back away from the battle at hand. It's okay if we lose a battle now and again. That's life. But too many battles lost will lose the war.

When we stop to look fear in the eye and push it aside to walk past it, it becomes a friend. When we face a fear or a problem, we're essentially smothering it and ourselves with love and light. Shedding light upon the darkness reveals the truth, and the truth is often simpler than we care to admit.

The Grand Canyon doesn't accept your troubles or excuses. Instead, it gives you the calculated adversity to help you eliminate those troubles yourself.

Like any good teacher, it doesn't heal you. It teaches you to heal yourself.

Epilogue

I had the chance to visit Lower Antelope Canyon a few years ago. In Page, Arizona. It's about 2 hours Northeast of the Grand Canyon I was both thrilled and disappointed.

I, like many, had been initiated into the twisted and magical slot canyons through the magic of the internet. More specifically, social media. I saw Instagram friends I had never met or known standing almost blissfully around the brown and red spiraling and twisted sandstone. The narrow walls make the scenery dramatic and inviting. In their photos, they seemed to be musing about solitude and wonder. Their heads were slightly tilted, with looks of contemplation on their faces, as if they were out for a casual stroll all by themselves and were caught unaware by a random photographer.

This was a place of beauty and peace. It was a place of awe and wonder. How could this place be a bad thing? Beauty, quiet contemplation, solitude, and awe? Sign me up.

So I went with a few friends and thought how great it would be to share the experience all alone with them in these majestic and sacred canyons. My perfect vision of the experience was based upon photos and emotions I had seen projected on Instagram.

Of course, my vision was wrong. I'll spare you every detail. But there were hundreds of people there clumped into groups of ten. We waited for the group in front to continue moving before we could access the path ahead. Photos were limited to a few seconds to prepare and shoot, and just like the Instagram photos, folks put on the "contemplative face" in order to get the photo they wanted in the three seconds they had to do it. They did this over and over again at every chance. The focus was them, not the beautiful canyon around them.

After being herded through and out like cattle, we tipped our required hired guide and moved on, wiser for the experience. Breathtaking canyon. In some ways, a disappointing experience.

Nature now often takes a back seat to the humans. People are no longer connected to the experience; they're connected to the validation and attention it brings them.

I hope that places like the Grand Canyon never become this bad, where the selfie is king. People no longer wanting a photo of the grandest place on Earth, simply wanting to indulge in their selfies. I hope the focus always remains on the beauty of the landscape.

We often look to our parents as heroes. There comes a sort of weird time when we realize that they are indeed human. They never let on, but they worried about making rent payments and raising children correctly, and they were trying to figure out life themselves. As we mature, there comes another wonderful time when our parents become more like friends in addition to being role models. The conversations are two-way. The laughs come easier. There's an understanding that we have all grown and grown up in the process.

My most recent visit to the Canyon felt like that. It was in the winter of 2020, about four months after I had hiked it. I went back to simply reminisce. To say hello.

The big, bad Canyon still inspired, but it was no longer as big or as bad. We had bonded and become friends. There were some things I almost felt like I could teach the Grand Canyon this time.

And just as a parent grows older, and roles from parent to child change, it was the same here. I offered information and tips to some visitors. Collected trash when I saw it. Smiled often to the passersby. The Canyon had taken such good care of me, I wanted to care for it back the best way I knew how.

I had hiked to the bottom, and now the Canyon and I were better friends.

I just wanted to be in the moment on this trip, absorbing all that the Canyon is. No expectations. Many times, I wandered along the rim trail, leaving the crowds behind. I would comfortably sit, perched safely near the rim, and listen. Just listen and observe.

Beyond the tourist aspect of the sights and conveniences of taking care of the masses and the tourists who come from all over the world, there lies a magic if you just sit long enough and listen for it. Luckily, many still do.

It has enthralled and enticed millions of visitors, artists, and thinkers for centuries. The Native Americans called both the rim and Canyon home. It was sacred ground to them.

Man has capitalized on and attempted to conquer the Canyon with little luck. It enchants and ensnares countless people every year. The Canyon was here long before us and will continue to flourish long after we're gone

Acknowledgments

It's always hard to try and convey the gratitude one has for the support, friendship, and love that make up your tribe. So many people have been an important part of my growth and journey, not just on the trails, but in life.

I'd like to thank the following for their contributions in one way or another for being a part of this project and for making me a better me.

My Parents, Frank and Rachel

Cory Dupuis

Robert Johnson

Shaun Francis